Regular solutions for skin inflammation

Introduction

Skin inflammation is certainly not a solitary sickness, but instead a name for gathering of infections associated because of comparable side effects. Skin rashes and immune system problems can be portrayed along these lines.

Typically, dryness shows up on hands, elbows, feet, knees, and on the face. Rashes on tainted regions begin to tingle and turn out to be much more aggravated when scratched. This disease isn't irresistible, yet it is enduring.

In addition, its power might change during the life expectancy. A few kids might congest the sensitivity while others remain exceptionally helpless. The ebb and flow sickness can cause extra ailments. Side effects and force of skin irritation are intended for every patient.

There is an assortment of skin inflammation types. Other than the most well-known case, atopic dermatitis, there are around six other sicknesses variations, different in their techniques for treatment and secondary effects.

Every one of them ought to be related to the assistance of an expert to guarantee a particular methodology for each case. Atopic dermatitis is a most broadly spread a sort of infection. It is normal among youngsters and is frequently connected with asthma and roughage fever.

Different sorts can be set off by contact with an unfavorably susceptible substance, stress, inappropriate saturating, bug chomps, temperature moves, strain and, surprisingly, hereditary inclination.

Each case is different in its look and aftereffects. The main normal thing for them is that they are kinds of sore and dry skin that ought not to be damaged.

There is no single assessment in regards to the reason for dermatitis. As indicated by the most recent exploration, different sorts of disease are brought about by their various standards. Especially, for the offspring of dermatitis sick guardians, the likelihood of fostering the disease is a lot higher.

The gamble pairs in situations where the two guardians have the sickness. Other than that, an amazing rundown of outer sources can influence assemblages of weak individuals and trigger the aggravation.

Wellsprings of risk can be separated into inner and outside types. Allergenic synthetic substances, temperature, food, and residue can cause a skin transformation from outside, while stress and hormonal movements impact side effects from the inside.

Dermatitis is generally spread among youngsters. They are more challenging to deal with, too. As dermatitis is relieved by the assessment of causes, the interaction can be darkened with regard to a youngster.

For this situation, it is normal for adults to limit the contact of a weak youngster with a recognized rundown of triggers of dermatitis. One ought to focus on the time and circumstance in which a likely physical and mental pressure occurred.

Dermatitis is a particular kind of infection. For every individual, a wellspring of pollution is explicit, as well as where the rashes show up and their sort.

By the by, side effects might be something similar among various individuals, particularly for the situation where they are family members. Its primary side effect is tingling, and one likewise may encounter different signs, from somewhat disturbing to perilously irritating.

The subsequent case encourages an evil individual to scratch the contaminated piece of skin until it drains, and accordingly to demolish his/her condition of wellbeing. The sort of skin aggravation can shift. Tingling and aggravation either vanish absolutely or return each instance of contact with the undesired matter.

It is enthusiastically prescribed to visit a nearby specialist to recognize a dermatitis type and consequently to settle on strategies for its treatment.

Ordinary treatment of dermatitis incorporates a blend of fundamental advances coordinated to balance out the state of the patient and limit the impact of disease on the human body. This disease is made essentially by a particularly unfavorably susceptible response to an outside trigger.

The initial step for every individual is subsequently to distinguish what is causing their sickness and limit superfluous cooperation with it. One likewise ought to stay away from the utilization of substances known as conceivable dermatitis triggers.

Besides, it is enthusiastically prescribed to take exceptional consideration for yourself; explicitly, to humidify the skin, keep away from distressing circumstances and abstain from scratching. Cures can likewise be utilized by the circumstance to limit the irritation.

Anti-microbial are applied to safeguard people in instances of outrageous skin diseases. Allergy meds work for counteraction and help with lessening tingling. The corticosteroid-comprehensive medications can be separated into ones for inside and outer use.

The outer use, for this situation, is profoundly liked, while the inward use brings about various aftereffects and ought to be utilized exclusively in instances of crisis. With specific kinds of dermatitis, immunomodulators and wet dressing can be utilized as well.

Simultaneously, an absence of fix managed the cost of by customary medication encouraged society to address a characteristic treatment of this sickness. In specific cases, long haul homeopathy treatment can turn out to be more useful while assuming a lesser measure of incidental effects.

Such methodology assesses the character of a patient, his inclinations, mental state, and even family issues. There are various results of day-to-day utilization that may decidedly impact the movement of the illness. They incorporate kimchee, rice, soybean food, and oat.

Extra nourishment with nutrients B, D and E and utilization of iodine-comprehensive food can likewise be helpful. Explicit washing fixings limit the gamble of irritation by water. In exceptional cases, probiotics decidedly affect the condition.

Other than that, different home-made recipes spin around skin saturating. Dermatitis chiefly upsets the skin's course of self-stuffing and self-dampening so one might utilize different oils to reproduce the equilibrium.

Dermatitis can't be restored. However, it tends to be taken care of to the degree that one scarcely sees the side effects. For each individual, there is the inward trigger that makes a sickness dynamic; distinguishing the reason might aid taking care of oneself.

The progression of sickness is an additional person. Simultaneously, there is no single assessment with respect to the methods of taking care of oneself, as both conventional and regular medication have their own solid and weak sides. As a rule, dermatitis can be taken care of under the condition that a wellspring of skin irritation is inaccessible.

Kinds of skin inflammation

Do you have any idea about which kind of skin inflammation you have? There are many sorts of dermatitis and those with one kind of skin inflammation will generally get another. A portion of the primary types of dermatitis are recorded here.

Atopic Dermatitis

You are brought into the world with a hereditary propensity to create atopic skin inflammation, yet the climate can likewise be a potential reason. It is an indication of an overactive resistant framework.

It is most normal in youngsters and signs appear inside the early long periods of life. A greater part will outgrow this by pubescence.

Atopic dermatitis is turning out to be progressively normal. Measurements for the Assembled Realm alone show us that offspring of young make up to 20 percent and grown-ups up to 5 percent of all atopic skin inflammation victims.

For this situation, the body produces huge amounts of the protein, which is a protein that follows up in the interest of the defensive cells of the resistant framework. It causes unfavorably susceptible responses.

We as a whole have this protein however with atopic dermatitis, significantly more is delivered because of the uplifted aversion to specific substances either by contact, by devouring specific food varieties and liquids and by inward breath and breathing airborne particles.

The issue is because of the resistant framework being overactive, which prompts irritation of the skin. With atopic dermatitis, you might foster aggravation contact skin inflammation also and be inclined toward roughage fever and asthma.

The most widely recognized allergens found in those with atopic dermatitis are house dust vermin or kissing bugs as they are better known, dust, pet skin and quills.

Different allergens incorporate yeasts found on the body and food sources like cow's milk, soya, wheat, nuts and eggs.

In a perfect world, figure out what you are sensitive to and keep away from it no matter what. Have a blood test to assist with diagnosing causes.

Flareups will show themselves as dry hot and irritated skin around the neck, knees, wrists, face and eyelids.

Asteatotic Skin inflammation

More normal in more seasoned individuals, ordinarily found on the leg, it brings about a red bothersome appearance.

Discoid Dermatitis

All age ranges will generally experience the ill effects of discoid dermatitis, however, it is tracked down fundamentally in more seasoned men. Grown-ups will more often than not respond to pressure and liquor in abundance. In kids and more youthful individuals, it is normal in those with a propensity to atopic dermatitis.

Seborrhoeic Dermatitis

Mostly found in grown-ups where there are enormous areas of sweat organs in the body. It is brought about by a lot of pityrosporum, which is an innocuous yeast shaped in the body. An enemy of yeast treatment will help.

It is tracked down chiefly on the scalp, face, armpits and crotch because of the bigger number of oil organs. The condition can differ from gentle where there is flaky skin to serious, where the skin becomes bothersome, sleek and kindled.

For scalp issues, hostile to yeast shampoos can assist with controlling it. For extreme cases, coal tar shampoos and selenium shampoos are frequently utilized.

Children are inclined to this type of dermatitis as a support cap on the scalp and the folds of the skin. As their skin is so fragile, you should make certain of the items utilized. A few suggested items incorporate emollient creams, antifungal creams, and steroid creams.

Fluid cream blended in with salicylic corrosive can assist with relaxing hard scaling from support cap. Wash this out a while later with cleanser explicitly for your child. A characteristic option is to rub olive oil on the scalp. This is a conventional cure that has been around for quite a long time.

Aggravation Contact Skin inflammation

This is extremely normal and is caused when there is contact with a substance that triggers extreme touchiness, followed by a hypersensitive response, because of the skin being disturbed.

Those with occupations that require the hands to get wet more than once, for example, beauticians, food laborers, cleaners, those that handle food, attendants and wellbeing laborers are the principal bunches who experience the ill effects of aggravation contact skin inflammation.

This is because of steady contact with specific substances and synthetics found in ordinary items that we use around the house and in the work environment.

Around 85% of the guilty parties are cleanser, cleansers and food. Blanches, elastic, skin meds, styling synthetic compounds and aromas are especially normal causes alongside paints and numerous items utilized for create making like pastes.

It is ridiculous to attempt to keep away from a significant number of these issues, as they are in the work environment and ordinary undertakings, so utilizing defensive gloves is fitting. As the elastic in a large portion of these gloves can exacerbate it, you ought to utilize the gloves with cotton inners or purchase a different set of slim breathable cotton gloves to wear inside the elastic gloves. This will help and keep away from exorbitant perspiring too, which can happen while wearing the elastic gloves for quite a while and decrease the opportunity of an episode.

The appearance is equivalent to ordinary dermatitis, and it is dealt with equivalent to unfavorably susceptible contact skin inflammation. Keeping the hands saturated to try not to as much break and parting of the skin is significant. Attempt to find natural, synthetic free obstruction creams as steroid creams has been known to exacerbate dermatitis in certain individuals.

Unfavorably susceptible Contact Skin inflammation

You can have a fix test to decide potential causes on the off chance that you are inclined to any of these aggravation issues.

The resistant framework recognizes specific substances that touch the skin as an unfamiliar body and the skin responds to these. Side effects incorporate sobbing, tingling and redness on the skin surface. Side effects ordinarily happen around the quick area of contact and afterward spread as the invulnerable cells begin to go to work.

It is essential to notice the side effects at the beginning, as you can all the more likely decide the reason and keep away from it later on. There are items we use in our regular day-to-day existences that we know nothing about. Only a couple of these are recorded beneath, with an example of what they are utilized for.

Those you might know about:-

Nickel - gems, studs on pants, bra cuts, butterfly hoop backs

Plants - unfavorably susceptible responses brought about by contact and breathing as in roughage fever

Those you might not know about:

Elastic - a portion of our dress and shoes contain elastic and different synthetic compounds

Epoxy gums - leisure activity makes glues

Colophony - utilized for mortars

Paraphenylenediamine - a few henna items and hair colors that are dark

Potassium dichromate - cowhide items

Cetearyl liquor - emollient creams

Neomycin - anti-microbial

Fusidic corrosive - anti-microbial

Steroid creams - hydrocortisone

Lanolin - lotion

As you will see, fixings contained in the steroid creams and lotions used to treat dermatitis might themselves at any point be the reason for the skin response. Right now, the genuine treatment being utilized could be aggravating the issue rather than improving it.

You may likewise need to stay away from close contact
with any individual who has a mouth blister.

The Eating routine for Beating Dermatitis

You should allude to the "Food Pyramid" in any case. On the off chance that your dermatitis is set off by a lack of stomach related, the accompanying regular dietary arrangement will monitor it. As per my experience, there have been cases in which these kinds of dermatitis victims even profess to have tracked down a remedy for their condition, so there is 100% expectation for you with it.

Regardless of whether your triggers come from food inadequacy, your dermatitis will be incredibly improved assuming that you apply the accompanying food routine. This regular enemy of dermatitis diet plan will work for anyone who isn't easily affected by the food sources which create it.

Nature Diet:- Fundamental Rules

From the food pyramid we as a whole know, I will be letting you know what sort of food sources you can eat to finish:

Fats and sugars:- The main fats we will consume will come as olive oil, whether it is utilized for searing (in its soaked structure), in plates of mixed greens, or from our wellspring of creature protein.

Dispense sugar prior to doing the eating routine we won't take Sugar. The thing we can take is honey (these contain additives and added sugars).

We will utilize 100% regular honey, which is effectively accessible in home-grown shops. As I have previously told you, disregard some other "honey" you can track down in the store. We will likewise take the sugar as fructose that the organic product contains normally.

Dairy items:- totally none.

Creature protein:- A chicken-based diet. No egg, no pork, no red meat, the equivalent goes for veal, every so often some salmon (an incredible Omega-3 source).

Differed Vegetables:- We can take a wide range of vegetables in pungent stews or anything that you like. One thing to remember isn't to involve vinegar in plates of mixed greens. No peculiar sauces either (in a couple of lines, I'll discuss what we can't have).

Organic products:- Take something like three bits of any natural product daily, assuming they are cleaned, much better. In any case, be exceptionally cautious with sensitivities. For instance, I can't eat bananas or pineapples since they give me sensitivities. I likewise don't suggest taking them before sleep time, particularly assuming that they are acidic.

Vegetables:- We can have chickpeas, lentils, and beans. I've attempted these and I haven't had any issues.

Dried organic products:- individuals with gastrointestinal lacks can't take them, as they can cause awful digestive agonies. Along these lines, I suggest you keep away from them on the off chance that this is your case.

Sugar:- Rice and just rice, entire grain and seed solely (both blended and entire grain as it were). Disallowed are bread and flours, regardless of whether they're rice-based flours or rice-based cakes and baked goods. No rice glues. We can have bubbled rice and stew. This will be our main Wellspring of Carbs.

Individuals under treatment for the most part do it with 50% entire grain and just seed. The admission of hydrates is vital, so you are permitted a great deal of rice in your feasts. The beneficial thing about rice is that it has numerous culinary conceivable outcomes. No potato or oat is practically identical to rice's flexibility. Along these lines, for this diet, you can't approach any cereal from rice; nothing will supplant it, no corn, just entire grain rice.

Everything can be decreased to organic products, oil, chicken, Vegetables, rice and honey (the last option in balance, a lot of honey can prompt weight stomach issues and weight gain, 2 - 3 tablespoons daily is the suggested portion).

Your favored implantations will be the matching supplement for this eating regimen, additionally consistently with honey and with practically no counterfeit flavors added. It's obviously true that imbuements are a compelling guide in the stomach related process.

Indeed, this is all there is to it for the rules, however for a more profound comprehension, I will give a few light notes.
Follow this:- We are not permitted to take any cakes or whatever contains flour of any sort.

We are not permitted to take whatever isn't on the past rundown, or that contains any sauces, from which we don't have the foggiest idea about the beginning.

We are not permitted to take any pre-prepared food

We are not permitted to drink any soft drinks or squeezes bought in business stores. Yet we can make imbuement with honey and ice which are flavorful!

We are not permitted to drink liquor of any sort. We should accept exceptional consideration with aged beverages like lager, wine, juice, and so on. We should not accept vinegar or whatever contains liquor to any degree, like olives, gherkins, and so forth.

This isn't expected to limit your get-together, worry won't as well. If you at any point hope to have a beverage, have a decent brand of rum on that extraordinary occasion (one of those that cost a larger number of than $36 a jug, please!), and you will not have any issue. Continuously have it with some restraint and return to your skin inflammation free eating regimen!

We can't believe everything that the servers in bars or cafés say to us. Recall that we can take Natural products, oil, vegetables, chicken, rice and honey.

For instance, in the event that we have a chicken stew in a bar and it has flour in it, the eating routine will be pointless.

-We are not permitted to take ketchup or seared tomatoes; to take broiled tomatoes, we can purchase filtered tomatoes without any added substances (it is inescapable that it has some, yet all the same minimizing would be ideal). We add somewhat salt and pepper oil, put it in the miniature 10 minutes to medium power and a choice broiled tomato will emerge.

We are not permitted to take any desserts regardless of whether they are without sugar, gum or any such thing. We are not permitted to have any sack of bites. We are not permitted to have espresso. We are not permitted to take any hotdog, totally none. No chicken frankfurters by the same token. (Take a gander at the fixings and you'll be stunned at how minimal chicken you have in there. Such a trick!).

We can't have anything we haven't cooked ourselves. Thus, adhere to the fixings rundown of the pyramid that Indeed, we can take toward the start of this demonstrated normal eating regimen way to deal with beat dermatitis!

As may be obvious, the eating routine is focused, which makes it exceptionally severe. Be that as it may, I urge you to disclose why and how many individuals stick to it. They are people who might have done anything. They would have favored anything in a genuine sense to having a body loaded with wounds. That is the quality and level of the mending power this beautiful eating routine arrangement has, and you will have it completely shown on the following page!

Aside from the eating regimen, it is Strongly Prescribed to take any nutrient enhancement liberated from flour or yeast. A few people take Solgar Recipe VM-75.

At long last, we should take a probiotic called "Saccharomyces boulardii" sold by numerous reasonable organizations like "Presently Food sources" or Jarrow Equations. However, not a medication, the main probiotic has been demonstrated to have the option to keep the stomach corrosive boundary alive.

After supper, take a portion of a level spoonful of baking pop. It ought to be noticed that bicarbonate gives sodium (salt) to our eating regimen, and the suggested everyday portion is 2.5 grams day to day, so we ought to bring down the portion of salt in our feasts.

In only 15 days, you ought to begin seeing an extreme improvement in your dermatitis; that is the manner by which strong this dinner plan is! As you will see without help from anyone else, this all around planned diet can contend and beat any substance based medicines, customary or elective.

I would say, this is the most reliable dietary strategy, the one device your body is yearning for, which has changed the existences of thousands of individuals. It awards ideal control of your dermatitis and conveys a progressive ability to mend your flare-ups.

It requires no unique elaboration. Simply adhere to the past proposals and you will actually want to plan what your body needs for getting recuperated. The eating regimen goes as follows, and you can go differing as per the pyramid rules. Simply go.

Normal Cures

Avocado and Aloe Vera Cover

This cover can be utilized on the face to ease dermatitis side effects, or as a glue on other impacted region of the body.

One avocado, pounded

One-tablespoon aloe vera gel
Combine fixings as one in a little bowl. Apply topically to the face or to different region of the body. Leave on for twenty minutes, and afterward flush with warm water and Dry.

Coconut Oil Cream

This straightforward as can be coconut oil cream has an extremely lengthy timeframe for realistic usability. Make a full clump and apply on a case-by-case basis, as your essential facial and body cream.

One cup crude coconut oil Two drops calendula rejuvenating ointment Combine fixings as one in a container. Apply to face and body as your ordinary lotion. Keep coconut oil cream fixed in a container while not being used.

Cereal Shower Splash

Utilize this alleviating oats to shower absorb by drifting the sack your shower, and tenderly scour your whole body with it.

One cup affirmed gluten moved oats One nut-milk pack or cheesecloth Fill the nut-milk sack wlth oats or put oats in cheesecloth and seal top with an elastic band or string.

Olive Leaf Ointment

For dermatitis that requirements broadened recuperating, apply this olive leaf treatment during the day or night, and cover with gloves or dress to keep the region secured.

Half cup unadulterated shea margarine Two drops olive leaf remove combine fixings as one in a container. Apply depending on the situation, as a balm, to impacted regions on the body and face.

Apricot Part Oil Saturating Cream

Utilize this delicate recuperating cream on the face or body. It has an unobtrusive smell and feels debauchedly smooth.

Half cup crude cocoa spread

One-quarter cup crude apricot piece oil One-quarter cup raw neem oil
Blend all fixings in with a blender, food processor, or hand blender. Place in a fixed container until prepared to utilize.

Olive Oil and Lavender Back rub Oil

There is something about lavender that appears to relieve the soul, which assists with mitigating the actual body, too. Rub a liberal measure of this olive oil and lavender back rub oil on impacted regions, or on your whole body, before you nod off around evening time.

One cup raw olive oil

Two drops of lavender rejuvenating oil blend fixings in a container. Keep fixed between utilizes.

Avocado Oil Cleanser

The way to getting a delicate fluid cleanser from this recipe is to begin with a totally unadulterated and plant-based cleanser bar. Search for one with coconut oil, hemp, or another vegetable oil base that is totally normal.

One four-ounce bar of normal cleanser
One-gallon water

Half cup raw avocado oil
Grind whole cleanser bar with a cheddar grater. Put away Heat water to the point of boiling. Eliminate from heat. Empty ground cleanser into the water and permit sitting for fifteen minutes. Mix with a hand blender until velvety. Add avocado oil and keep on mixing for one more moment. Permit cooling. Fill a holder with a siphon to utilize.

Delicate Face Cleaning agent

This delicate face cleaning agent is normal and extraordinary for relieving irritation.

One-tablespoon crude honey

One-tablespoon plain soy or coconut milk yogurt One teaspoon dangerous elm, dried and powdered blend fixings and apply to confront. Delicately focus on whole face round movements for twenty seconds. Flush with warm water and dry.

Turmeric Tea

This skin inflammation recipe begins adjusting the body inside so you can get the advantages of outside mending.

Two cups of separated water

One-teaspoon ground turmeric One-teaspoon crude honey

One cut lemon

Carry water to a delicate bubble. Add turmeric and permit soaking for five to ten minutes. Add honey and lemon to taste. Appreciate.

Stinging Bramble Tea

Recuperating is an inside work, yet this stinging weed tea performs twofold responsibility when consumed day to day and utilized as a relieving skin treatment for the skin.

Four cups separated water

Four tablespoons stinging weed tea Four tablespoons crude honey
Carry water to a delicate bubble. Add stinging weed leaves and permit soaking for five to ten minutes. Add honey. Drink some the tea every day and plunge a washcloth in leftover tea to apply every day to impacted regions. Don't bother flushing.

Conclusion

Albeit the reason for dermatitis stays unclear, it's obviously true that contamination, in the mix of hereditary legacy are demonstrated significant causes, which influence our safe framework which considers our skin.

For the world outside, the inherence of ecological specialists is a reason for the dermatitis condition. It is fundamental to establish cognizance towards saving our current circumstance from contamination and keep away from the different ecological elements that might be at the foundation of atopic dermatitis.

Limiting openness to ecological allergens, unforgiving cleansers, cleansers, and unexpected changes in temperature and lessening anxiety have been shown to be useful for most dermatitis patients.

Through better information on your condition, you will actually want to foster that impulse that will direct you to pick the food varieties and activities your body expects to mend. Information is the key; information on you and your circumstances. The eating routine and recipes introduced can and ought to be changed, keeping the key fixings, or reciprocals, in the core of every recipe.

Long-lasting hydration and omega-3 and 6 supplementations are the favored arrangements among devotees of normal solutions for skin inflammation. Ongoing logical exploration appears to support the possibility that skin inflammation can for sure be effectively treated with omega-3 and 6.

Through this extreme and disclosing venture, I have given you rule, realities and cures that will tune you in to the correct way towards overseeing dermatitis. Likewise, I want to believe that you will foster a more profound degree of cognizance to direct your recharged life and activities better.

By changing your propensities and reflecting while at the same time applying the information in this book, you will get to realize yourself better. That is the lovely gift normal methodology generally conveys to the man of harmony.